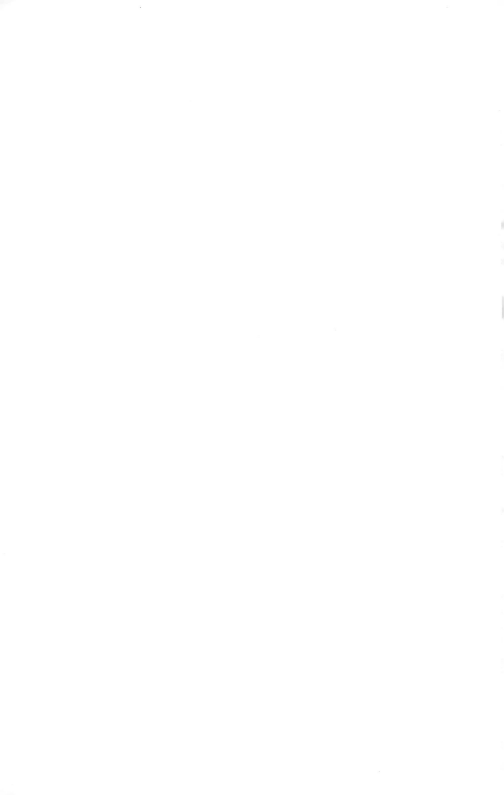

Labs & Imaging for Primary Eye Care

Optometry In Full Scope

The Fine Art of Patient Management

John R Martinelli MD OD FAAO

OPHTHALMIC PHYSICIAN PUBLISHING
Sharing The Fine Art of Patient Management

For Melissa...

Contents

Medical Disclaimer   vii

Introduction   ix

HIGH-YIELD LABS FOR PRIMARY
EYE CARE   1

Complete Blood Count with Differential
(CBC w/diff)   1

Comprehensive Metabolic Profile (CMP)   4

Fasting Blood Glucose (FBG) and
Glycosylated Hemoglobin (HbA1C
or A1C)   7

Erythrocyte Sedimentation Rate (ESR)   9

C-Reactive Protein (CRP)   11

Antinuclear Antibody (ANA)   13

Rheumatoid Factor (RF)   16

HLA-B27   19

Lipid Profile   21

aPTT (Activated Partial Thromboplastin
Time)   23

PT (Prothrombin Time)   25

International Normalized Ratio (INR)   26

Thyroid Function Tests (TFT)   29

HIGH-YIELD IMAGING FOR PRIMARY
EYE CARE   31

Computed Tomography (CT) Head
and/or Orbits   31

CT Angiography (CTA)   34

CT with Contrast vs CTA   35

Magnetic Resonance Imaging (MRI)
Brain and/or Orbits   39

Magnetic Resonance Angiography (MRA)   42
Magnetic Resonance Venography (MRV)   44
FIESTA Protocol MRI   46
Echocardiogram (Echo)   49
Carotid Duplex or Doppler Ultrasound   51

ELECTRODIAGNOSTIC INVESTIGATIONS   54
Electrocardiogram (ECG/EKG)   54
Electroencephalogram (EEG)   56
Visual Evoked Potentials (VEP)   59
Electroretinogram (ERG)   61

WRITING THE SCRIPTS   65
Steps for Writing an Order: 65

LOGISTICS   68

Conclusion   71
Resources   73
Test Your Knowledge   85
Answers   93
About the Author   99

Medical Disclaimer

Please note the information contained within this book is for educational purposes only. All effort has been executed to present accurate, up-to-date, reliable, complete information. The content within this book has been derived from various sources. Please consult a licensed physician before implementing diagnostic methods and/or treatments outlined in this book.

By reading this book, the reader agrees that under no circumstances is the author responsible for any losses, direct or indirect, that are incurred because of the use of the information contained within this book, including, but not limited to, errors, omissions, or inaccuracies.

Please note the information provided below is for general informational purposes. It is not intended to diagnose, treat, cure, or prevent any disease, and it should not be relied upon as a substitute for consultations with qualified healthcare professionals.

Ophthalmic Physician Publishing strives to ensure the information presented is accurate and up to date, but we make no representations or warranties of any kind, express or implied, about the completeness, accuracy, reliability, suitability, or availability with respect to the information provided. Any reliance you place on such information is strictly at your own risk.

Introduction

Welcome to Labs and Imaging for Primary Eye Care

Optometry has evolved significantly over the past century, with a core philosophy of providing comprehensive medical eye care that addresses the needs of the entire individual. After decades of advocacy and educational advancements, the practice of optometry in the United States now faces minimal restrictions, allowing you to offer a broad and complete scope of care.

The goal of this book is to guide you and provide practical insights, helping you align your practice within the scope of medicine.

What This Book Is

This book serves as a straightforward and fundamental guide to help you understand and efficiently order labs and imaging diagnostics. By becoming more comfortable with these investigations, you will be better equipped to make informed decisions in managing your patients effectively.

What This Book Is Not

This book is not intended to be an instructional on interpreting laboratory or imaging results. Short examples are given; however, interpretation skills are developed through continuous study and patient interactions, positioning yourself correctly in practice, and gaining appropriate experience.

Yours For The Taking

A multitude of diagnostic investigations are available and within your scope of practice to order. Utilizing these resources responsibly and effectively is required for providing comprehensive patient care. Deciding where to begin and determining the most appropriate orders can be challenging, even for seasoned clinicians.

As an optometrist, you work within a defined specialty where certain labs and imaging can be commonly ordered, forming your "usual formulary" and comfort zone. However, there will be occasions when you need to step outside this comfort zone to provide the best care for your patients. For example, obtaining a lumbar puncture for an optic neuritis patient with an unremarkable brain MRI, to differentiate between an inflammatory or infectious source.

Approaching Diagnostics Empathetically

When ordering labs and imaging, it is important to approach this higher level of diagnostics empathetically. Remember, your patients are real people who are often anxious for results and solutions to their problems. At this level, time consciousness regarding results and communication is always a priority.

Also consider, pursuing an underlying etiology or source of a problem is sometimes more than a priority; it is an urgency. It can be the difference between stroke or no stroke, paralysis or no paralysis, heart attack or no heart attack, loss of vision or no loss of vision, death or no death. When an individual is in your chair, you must take responsibility to recognize the issue at hand and manage it promptly.

Minimizing Unnecessary Referrals

Unnecessary referrals often waste precious time and create greater anxiety and distress for your patients. Your proper management will eliminate the involvement of additional medical personnel, resources, energy, time, money, and insurance burden. And, you might just save a life or major debilitating consequences by saving time.

Embracing Your Primary Care Role

Embracing your primary care role, which includes laboratory medicine and imaging as part of your daily practice, is essential for you and your patients. Additionally, the specialty of optometry is elevated and more properly recognized within the medical community.

———————

High-Yield Labs for Primary Eye Care

Complete Blood Count with Differential (CBC w/diff)

A Complete Blood Count (CBC) is a comprehensive investigation which evaluates various blood components, including leukocytes or white blood cells (WBC's), red blood cells (RBC's), hemoglobin (HGB), hematocrit (HCT), and platelets. This is important for diagnosing a range of conditions and can reveal multiple illnesses which may be characterized and discovered in blood. Examples include forms of anemia, inflammation, allergy, infection, leukemia, lymphoma, and many others.

A CBC *without differential* measures the number of platelets, red and white blood cells, along with hemoglobin and hematocrit values. Red blood cell indices such as mean corpuscle volume (MCV), mean corpuscular hemoglobin (MCH), and mean corpuscular hemoglobin concentration (MCHC) describe the volume of red blood cells and their hemoglobin content. These are reported along with the red blood cell distribution width (RDW), which measures the variation in the sizes of red blood cells.

A CBC *with differential* provides additional information enumerating the various types of WBC's, and also includes a count of immature RBC's or reticulocytes. This differential which is usually ordered as part of the CBC, indicates specific levels of the five white blood cell types and includes neutrophils, lymphocytes, monocytes, eosinophils and basophils, as well as abnormal cell types present. Results are reported as percentages and absolute values, then compared against reference ranges to determine whether the values are normal, low, or high.

Normal CBC w/diff Values:

- **WBC**: 4500-11000 cells/mcL
- **RBC**: 4.5-6.0 million cells/mcL (men), 4.0-5.5 million cells/mcL (women)
- **Hemoglobin**: 13.8-17.2 g/dL (men), 12.1-15.1 g/dL (women)
- **Hematocrit**: 40-52% (men), 35-47% (women)
- **Platelets**: 150,000-450,000 cells/mcL

Interpretation of CBC Values:

- **High WBC**: Suggestive of infection, inflammation, or hematologic malignancy like leukemia.
- **Low WBC**: May indicate bone marrow suppression, autoimmune disease, or severe infection.
- **High RBC, Hemoglobin, Hematocrit**: Can be due to polycythemia or dehydration.
- **Low RBC, Hemoglobin, Hematocrit**: Indicative of anemia or blood loss.
- **High Platelets**: Often seen in inflammatory states or bone marrow disorders.
- **Low Platelets**: Can point to bleeding disorders or bone marrow failure.

Example Cases:

Case 1: Anemia

- **Presentation**: A patient with fatigue, pallor, and shortness of breath.
- **Lab Results**: Hemoglobin: 10.5 g/dL (low), Hematocrit: 32% (low), MCV: 75 fL (low).
- **Management**: Consider iron supplements if iron deficiency is confirmed or further investigations for other causes of anemia.

Case 2: Leukemia

- **Presentation**: A patient with frequent infection, bruising, and fatigue.

- **Lab Results**: WBC: 50,000 cells/mcL (high) with the presence of blast cells.
- **Management**: Urgent referral to hematology/oncology for further evaluation and treatment.

Case 3: Thrombocytopenia

- **Presentation**: A patient with petechiae, easy bruising, and nosebleeds.
- **Lab Results**: Platelets: 80,000 cells/mcL (low).
- **Management**: Investigate underlying causes (e.g., autoimmune conditions, medications) and manage accordingly, possibly involving a hematology consultation.

Comprehensive Metabolic Profile (CMP)

Also known as a metabolic panel, SMA-12+2, chem 14, chemistry panel, or chemistry screen.

The CMP is an extensive panel assessing hepatic and renal function, electrolyte levels, and glucose levels. It is an expanded version of the basic metabolic panel (BMP) which does not include liver enzymes and function. This panel of 14 components in blood serves as an initial broad medical screening tool, and also provides parathyroid status (Ca levels) as well as information to assess acid/base and fluid/blood volume balance.

Components of CMP:

- **Glucose**: 70-99 mg/dL (fasting)
- **Calcium**: 8.5-10.2 mg/dL
- **Albumin**: 3.5-5.0 g/dL
- **Total Protein**: 6.0-8.3 g/dL
- **Sodium**: 135-145 mEq/L
- **Potassium**: 3.5-5.0 mEq/L
- **CO2 (Bicarbonate)**: 23-29 mEq/L
- **Chloride**: 96-106 mEq/L
- **Blood Urea Nitrogen (BUN)**: 7-20 mg/dL
- **Creatinine**: 0.6-1.2 mg/dL
- **ALP (Alkaline Phosphatase)**: 44-147 IU/L
- **ALT (Alanine Aminotransferase)**: 7-56 IU/L
- **AST (Aspartate Aminotransferase)**: 10-40 IU/L
- **Bilirubin**: 0.1-1.2 mg/dL

Interpretation of CMP Values:

- **High Glucose**: Suggests diabetes or stress response.
- **Low Glucose**: Can indicate hypoglycemia, possibly due to insulin overdose, fasting, or adrenal insufficiency.
- **High Calcium**: May be due to hyperparathyroidism, malignancy, or excessive vitamin D intake.
- **Low Calcium**: Can be caused by hypoparathyroidism, vitamin D deficiency, or renal failure.

- **High/Low Sodium**: Indicative of dehydration, kidney dysfunction, or adrenal gland problems.
- **High/Low Potassium**: Can be due to kidney disease, adrenal issues, or effects of medications.
- **High BUN/Creatinine**: Indicates potential kidney dysfunction or dehydration.
- **High ALP, ALT, AST, Bilirubin**: Suggests liver disease, bile duct obstruction, or hepatitis.

Example Cases:

Case 1: Diabetes

- **Presentation**: A patient with increased thirst, frequent urination, and unexplained weight loss.
- **Lab Results**: Glucose: 150 mg/dL (high).
- **Management**: Lifestyle modifications, blood glucose monitoring, and possibly starting diabetes medication.

Case 2: Liver Disease

- **Presentation**: A patient with jaundice, abdominal pain, and fatigue.
- **Lab Results**: ALT: 120 IU/L (high), AST: 90 IU/L (high), Bilirubin: 2.5 mg/dL (high).

- **Management**: Further evaluation for liver disease, including imaging and possible referral to hepatology.

Case 3: Kidney Dysfunction

- **Presentation**: A patient with swelling in the legs, fatigue, and high blood pressure.
- **Lab Results**: BUN: 35 mg/dL (high), Creatinine: 2.0 mg/dL (high).
- **Management**: Manage underlying conditions, dietary changes, and possible referral to nephrology.

Fasting Blood Glucose (FBG) and Glycosylated Hemoglobin (HbA1C or A1C)

FBG measures serum glucose levels after an overnight fast, while HbA1c provides average blood glucose levels over approximately 90 days.

A1C measures the percentage of hemoglobin that has glucose attached to it. When glucose is present in the bloodstream, it attaches to hemoglobin in RBC's through a process known as glycosylation. Since RBC's have a lifespan of about 120 days, the A1C reflects the average blood glucose levels over the previous two to three months. Therefore, the higher the blood glucose levels, the greater the amount of glycosylated hemoglobin. This long-term indicator provides a more comprehensive picture of glucose levels and control compared to daily blood glucose.

The convenience of the A1C lies in its simplicity, as it requires just a single blood sample that can be taken at any time of day without the need for fasting.

Fasting Blood Glucose:

- **Normal Values**: 70-99 mg/dL
- **Prediabetes**: 100-125 mg/dL
- **Diabetes**: ≥126 mg/dL

Hemoglobin A1C (HbA1c):

- **Normal Values**: <5.7%
- **Prediabetes**: 5.7-6.4%
- **Diabetes**: ≥6.5%

Example Cases:

Case 1: Diabetes Diagnosis

- **Presentation**: A patient with increased thirst, frequent urination, and unexplained weight loss.
- **Lab Results**: Fasting Blood Glucose: 150 mg/dL (high), HbA1c: 7.5% (high).
- **Management**: Lifestyle modifications, blood glucose monitoring, and initiation of diabetes medication.

Case 2: Prediabetes Management

- **Presentation**: A patient with a family history of diabetes and mild symptoms like fatigue.
- **Lab Results**: Fasting Blood Glucose: 110 mg/dL (prediabetes), HbA1c: 6.0% (prediabetes).
- **Management**: Lifestyle changes including diet and exercise, and regular monitoring of blood glucose levels.

Case 3: Poor Glycemic Control in Known Diabetic

- **Presentation**: A known diabetic patient with signs of poor glycemic control, such as frequent infections.
- **Lab Results**: HbA1c: 9.0% (high).
- **Management**: Adjust current medication regimen, reinforce lifestyle changes, and consider insulin therapy if necessary.

Erythrocyte Sedimentation Rate (ESR)

Also known as an ESR or Sed Rate.

ESR is a measure of the rate at which red blood cells in anti-coagulated whole blood descend in a standardized tube over a period of one hour. Anti-coagulated blood is placed in an upright tube, known as a Westergren tube, and the distance at which the red blood cells fall is measured and reported in millimeters at the end of one hour.

It is a nonspecific marker of increased inflammation, pregnancy, anemia, autoimmune disorders such as rheumatoid arthritis and lupus, infection, certain renal disease, and some cancers including lymphoma and multiple myeloma.

Normal ESR Values:

- **Men**: <15 mm/hr or Age/2
- **Women**: <20 mm/hr or Age+10/2

Interpretation:

- **High ESR**: Suggestive of inflammatory conditions, autoimmune disease, infection, or malignancy.
- **Low ESR**: May be indicative of polycythemia, hyperviscosity syndromes, or sickle cell anemia.

Example Cases:

Case 1: Giant Cell Arteritis

- **Presentation**: A patient with headache, jaw claudication, and vision changes.
- **Lab Results**: ESR: 70 mm/hr (high).
- **Management**: Immediate initiation of corticosteroids and referral to rheumatology.

Case 2: Rheumatoid Arthritis

- **Presentation**: A patient with joint pain, stiffness, and swelling.
- **Lab Results**: ESR: 45 mm/hr (high).
- **Management**: Referral to rheumatology for further evaluation and management.

Case 3: Inflammatory Bowel Disease

- **Presentation**: A patient with abdominal pain, diarrhea, and weight loss.
- **Lab Results**: ESR: 50 mm/hr (high).
- **Management**: Referral to gastroenterology for further evaluation and management.

C-Reactive Protein (CRP)

This protein is an annular or ring-shaped pentameric protein found in blood plasma, whose circulating concentrations rise in response to inflammation. It is an acute-phase protein of hepatic origin that increases following interleukin-6 secretion by macrophages and T cells involved in the immune response. Its role is to bind to lysophosphatidylcholine expressed on the surface of dead or dying cells and some types of bacteria in order to activate the inflammatory cascade triggering the complement system.

Measuring and following CRP values can prove useful in determining disease progress in terms of waxing or waning as well as the effectiveness of treatments. Normal levels increase with aging. Higher levels can be found in late pregnant women, viral infection, bacterial infection, active inflammation, and burns.

CRP is a more sensitive and accurate measure of the acute phase inflammatory response than ESR. Therefore, in certain clinical scenarios, the ESR may be initially normal while CRP is elevated. CRP also returns to normal more quickly than ESR in response to treatment.

CRP Levels:

- **Low**: <1.0 mg/L
- **Average**: 1.0-3.0 mg/L
- **High**: >3.0 mg/L

Interpretation:

- **High CRP**: Indicates active inflammation, bacterial infection, or chronic inflammatory disease.
- **Low CRP**: Generally normal but can be seen in certain conditions with low inflammatory response.

Example Cases:

Case 1: Bacterial Infection

- **Presentation**: A patient with fever, chills, and body aches.
- **Lab Results**: CRP: 15 mg/L (high).
- **Management**: Prescribe antibiotics and monitor response to treatment.

Case 2: Rheumatoid Arthritis

- **Presentation**: A patient with joint pain, stiffness, and swelling.
- **Lab Results**: CRP: 8 mg/L (high).
- **Management**: Referral to rheumatology and initiate anti-inflammatory therapy.

Case 3: Inflammatory Bowel Disease

- **Presentation**: A patient with abdominal pain, diarrhea, and weight loss.
- **Lab Results**: CRP: 12 mg/L (high).
- **Management**: Referral to gastroenterology for further evaluation and treatment.

Antinuclear Antibody (ANA)

Also known as anti-nuclear factor, ANF, fluorescent anti-nuclear antibody test, FANA.

Antinuclear antibodies are auto-antibodies that bind to contents of the cell nucleus. In normal individuals, the immune system produces antibodies to foreign protein antigens but not to human proteins.

Antibodies targeting human antigens is an abnormal response and are known as auto-antigens

There are many sub-types of ANA's such as anti-R antibodies, anti-La antibodies, anti-Sm antibodies, anti-nRNP antibodies, anti-Scl-70 antibodies, anti-dsDNA antibodies, anti-histone antibodies, antibodies to nuclear pore complexes, anti-centromere antibodies and anti-sp100 antibodies. Each of these antibody subtypes binds to different proteins or protein complexes within the nucleus.

They are found in many disorders including autoimmunity, cancer, infection, with different prevalence's of auto-antibodies depending on the condition. Examples include systemic lupus erythematosus (SLE), rheumatoid arthritis (RA), sjögren syndrome, scleroderma, polymyositis, dermatomyositis, primary biliary cirrhosis, drug induced lupus, autoimmune hepatitis, multiple sclerosis, discoid lupus, certain thyroid disease, antiphospholipid syndrome (APS), juvenile rheumatoid arthritis (JRA), psoriatic arthritis (PsA), juvenile dermatomyositis, idiopathic thrombocytopenic purpura (ITP), and others.

These auto-antibodies can be subdivided according to their specificity, and each subset has different propensities for specific disorders. The pattern present under a fluorescent microscope gives additional clues as to an etiologic source. The lab report will give you this pattern to help guide and develop your working diagnosis.

Monitoring levels helps gauge the progression of disease. A positive ANA is most useful if associated clinical or laboratory data supporting a diagnosis are present.

ANA Patterns:

- **Homogeneous**: Common in systemic lupus erythematosus (SLE).
- **Speckled**: Seen in SLE, Sjögren's syndrome, scleroderma.
- **Nucleolar**: Seen in scleroderma and polymyositis.
- **Centromere**: Common in CREST syndrome.

Interpretation:

- **Positive ANA**: Suggests autoimmune disease but must be correlated with clinical findings.
- **Negative ANA**: Reduces likelihood of autoimmune disease but does not rule them out completely.

Example Cases:

Case 1: Systemic Lupus Erythematosus (SLE)

- **Presentation**: A patient with malar rash, joint pain, and fatigue.

- **Lab Results**: ANA: Positive Homogeneous pattern.
- **Management**: Referral to rheumatology for further evaluation and treatment.

Case 2: Sjögren's Syndrome

- **Presentation**: A patient with dry eyes, dry mouth, and joint pain.
- **Lab Results**: ANA: Positive Speckled pattern.
- **Management**: Referral to rheumatology and initiate symptomatic treatment for dryness.

Case 3: Scleroderma

- **Presentation**: A patient with skin thickening, Raynaud's phenomenon, and joint pain.
- **Lab Results**: ANA: Positive Nucleolar pattern.
- **Management**: Referral to rheumatology for further evaluation and management.

Rheumatoid Factor (RF)

Rheumatoid Factor is an autoantibody predominantly of the IgM class, but can also belong to other immunoglobulin classes like IgG, IgA, and IgE. It is directed against the Fc portion of IgG, forming immune complexes that contribute to the inflammatory response seen in autoimmune diseases. The RF test is primarily used in the diagnosis of Rheumatoid Arthritis (RA), an autoimmune condition characterized by chronic inflammation of synovial joints. However, elevated RF levels can also be found in other autoimmune disorders, chronic infections, and even in a subset of the healthy population, particularly the elderly, making its specificity a point of consideration in clinical interpretation.

The laboratory investigation for RF typically involves quantitative and qualitative assays, with the most commonly used methods being enzyme-linked immunosorbent assay (ELISA), nephelometry, and latex agglutination tests. Nephelometry and ELISA are highly sensitive and precise, offering quantitative results that help assess the disease severity and monitor treatment response. Latex agglutination, although less sensitive, remains a common rapid screening test. Elevated RF levels, especially when detected alongside other markers like anti-citrullinated protein antibodies (ACPA), strongly indicate the presence of RA, although not all patients with RA test positive for RF. Negative RF does not exclude the diagnosis, particularly in the early stages of RA or in seronegative variants of the condition.

RF Levels:

- **Negative**: <20 IU/mL
- **Positive**: >20 IU/mL

Interpretation:

- **Positive RF**: Suggestive of rheumatoid arthritis or other autoimmune disease.
- **Negative RF**: Does not rule out rheumatoid arthritis; further testing may be necessary.

Example Cases:

Case 1: Rheumatoid Arthritis

- **Presentation**: A patient with symmetrical joint pain, stiffness, and swelling.
- **Lab Results**: RF: 60 IU/mL (positive).
- **Management**: Referral to rheumatology for further evaluation and treatment with DMARDs.

Case 2: Sjögren's Syndrome

- **Presentation**: A patient with dry eyes, dry mouth, and joint pain.
- **Lab Results**: RF: 45 IU/mL (positive).
- **Management**: Referral to rheumatology and initiate symptomatic treatment for dryness.

Case 3: Hepatitis C

- **Presentation**: A patient with fatigue, jaundice, and joint pain.
- **Lab Results**: RF: 30 IU/mL (positive).
- **Management**: Referral to gastroenterology for further evaluation and antiviral therapy.

HLA-B27

Also known as human leukocyte antigen B27, human leukocyte A antigen, histocompatibility leukocyte A antigen.

HLA-B27 is known as a class I surface antigen encoded by the B locus in the major histocompatibility complex, MHC, on chromosome 6. This code allows for the production of antigenic cellular surface peptides derived from self and non-self triggers which are recognized by T cells. It is strongly associated with ankylosing spondylitis, however, it can also be a factor in other inflammatory disease, such as psoriatic arthritis, inflammatory bowel disease, and reactive arthritis.

The prevalence of HLA-B27 varies markedly in the global population. For example, about 8% of Caucasians, 4% of North Africans, 2–9% of Chinese, and 0.1–0.5% of persons of Japanese descent possess the gene that codes for this antigen. In Scandinavia, 24% of people are HLA-B27 positive, while only 1.8% have associated ankylosing spondylitis. In Finland, an estimated 14% of the population is positive for HLA-B27.

This relationship between HLA-B27 and many conditions continues to be investigated and studied. Though HLA-B27 is associated with a wide range of disease, it does not appear to be the sole mediator in development. It is however implicated in other types of seronegative (RA negative) spondyloarthropathy including reactive arthritis, anterior uveitis, psoriatic arthritis, Crohn's and ulcerative colitis. HLA antigens have also been implicated in autism.

HLA-B27 Presence:

- **Positive**: Indicates increased risk for certain autoimmune diseases.
- **Negative**: Does not rule out the diseases but lowers the probability.

Interpretation:

- **Positive HLA-B27**: Suggestive of conditions like ankylosing spondylitis, reactive arthritis, or anterior uveitis.
- **Negative HLA-B27**: Reduces the likelihood of these conditions but does not rule them out completely.

Example Cases:

Case 1: Ankylosing Spondylitis

- **Presentation**: A patient with chronic back pain and stiffness.
- **Lab Results**: HLA-B27: Positive.
- **Management**: Referral to rheumatology for further evaluation and initiation of appropriate therapy.

Case 2: Reactive Arthritis

- **Presentation**: A patient with joint pain following a gastrointestinal infection.
- **Lab Results**: HLA-B27: Positive.
- **Management**: Symptomatic treatment and referral to rheumatology if symptoms persist.

Case 3: Anterior Uveitis

- **Presentation**: A patient with eye pain, redness, and photophobia.
- **Lab Results**: HLA-B27: Positive.
- **Management**: Topical and/or oral steroids, topical cycloplegia.

Lipid Profile

Also known as a lipid panel, lipoprotein profile, coronary risk profile.

A lipid profile is a serologic assessment used to find abnormalities in lipids, which include various forms of cholesterol and triglycerides. The result can identify certain genetic disease and can determine approximate risk for cardiovascular disease, certain forms of pancreatitis, and other conditions. High levels of low density lipoproteins (LDL), very low density lipoproteins (VLDL), and total cholesterol increase the risk of cardiovascular disease and a host of vasculopathies. Low levels of protective high density lipoproteins (HDL) are also increase risk.

Components of Lipid Profile:

- **Total Cholesterol**: <200 mg/dL
- **HDL (High-Density Lipoprotein)**: >60 mg/dL
- **LDL (Low-Density Lipoprotein)**: <100 mg/dL
- **Triglycerides**: <150 mg/dL

Interpretation:

- **High Total Cholesterol/LDL**: Increased risk for cardiovascular disease.
- **Low HDL**: Increased risk for cardiovascular disease.
- **High Triglycerides**: Associated with increased risk of pancreatitis and cardiovascular disease.

Example Cases:

Case 1: Hyperlipidemia

- **Presentation**: A patient with a family history of heart disease and elevated cholesterol.
- **Lab Results**: Total Cholesterol: 250 mg/dL (high), LDL: 160 mg/dL (high), HDL: 40 mg/dL (low).
- **Management**: Lifestyle modifications and initiation of statin therapy.

Case 2: Cardiovascular Disease

- **Presentation**: A patient with chest pain and shortness of breath.
- **Lab Results**: Total Cholesterol: 220 mg/dL (high), LDL: 140 mg/dL (high), HDL: 35 mg/dL (low).
- **Management**: Referral to cardiology for further evaluation and management.

Case 3: Pancreatitis

- **Presentation**: A patient with severe abdominal pain and a history of alcohol use.
- **Lab Results**: Triglycerides: 500 mg/dL (high).
- **Management**: Hospitalization and initiation of treatment for pancreatitis.

aPTT (Activated Partial Thromboplastin Time)

Activated Partial Thromboplastin Time (aPTT) evaluates the intrinsic coagulation pathway by measuring the time it takes for blood to clot. Prolonged aPTT suggests bleeding disorders, and also found with heparin therapy, while shortened aPTT is less common but may indicate hypercoagulable states.

aPTT Levels:

- **Normal**: 25-35 seconds

Interpretation:

- **Prolonged aPTT**: Indicates potential bleeding disorders, factor deficiencies, or heparin therapy.
- **Shortened aPTT**: May indicate hypercoagulable states but is less common.

Example Cases:

Case 1: Hemophilia

- **Presentation**: A patient with spontaneous bleeding and bruising.
- **Lab Results**: aPTT: 60 seconds (prolonged).
- **Management**: Referral to hematology for further evaluation and factor replacement therapy.

Case 2: Heparin Therapy Monitoring

- **Presentation**: A patient on heparin therapy for deep vein thrombosis.
- **Lab Results**: aPTT: 70 seconds (prolonged).
- **Management**: Adjust heparin dosage to maintain therapeutic range.

Case 3: Liver Disease

- **Presentation**: A patient with jaundice and a history of alcohol abuse.
- **Lab Results**: aPTT: 55 seconds (prolonged).
- **Management**: Further evaluation for liver function and possible referral to hepatology.

PT (Prothrombin Time)

PT s a method for evaluating the extrinsic pathway and common pathway of coagulation. It is used to determine the clotting tendency of blood as well as a measure of hepatic disease (coagulation factors are produced in the liver). It measures the following coagulation factors: I (fibrinogen), II (prothrombin), V (proaccelerin), VII (proconvertin), and X (Stuart–Prower factor). Vitamin K levels and warfarin therapy can also be assessed providing essential information for managing coagulation disorders.

PT Levels:

- **Normal**: 11-13.5 seconds

Interpretation:

- **Prolonged PT**: Indicates potential liver disease, vitamin K deficiency, or warfarin therapy.
- **Shortened PT**: Less common, usually not clinically significant.

Example Cases:

Case 1: Vitamin K Deficiency

- **Presentation**: A patient with easy bruising and prolonged bleeding after minor cuts.
- **Lab Results**: PT: 20 seconds (prolonged).
- **Management**: Vitamin K supplementation and dietary advice.

Case 2: Warfarin Therapy Monitoring

- **Presentation**: A patient on warfarin therapy for atrial fibrillation.
- **Lab Results**: PT: 25 seconds (prolonged).
- **Management**: Adjust warfarin dosage to maintain therapeutic INR range.

Case 3: Liver Cirrhosis

- **Presentation**: A patient with jaundice, ascites, and history of chronic alcohol use.
- **Lab Results**: PT: 22 seconds (prolonged).
- **Management**: Referral to hepatology for further management of liver cirrhosis.

International Normalized Ratio (INR)

The INR is the ratio of an individuals prothrombin time to a normal control sample, raised to the power of the international sensitivity index (ISI) value for the analytical system being used.

The result in seconds for PT performed on a normal individual will vary according to the type of analytical system employed. This is due to the variations between different types and batches of manufacturer's tissue factor used in the reagent to perform the test. The INR was devised to standardize the results. Each manufacturer assigns an ISI value for any tissue factor they manufacture, which indicates how a particular type of tissue factor compares to the international reference.

The INR therefore standardizes PT results, primarily utilized for consistent management of individuals on warfarin therapy. High INR indicates an increased risk of bleeding, while low INR suggests a risk of clotting. Maintaining INR within the targeted therapeutic range is critical for patients on anticoagulation therapy.

INR Levels:

- **Normal:** 0.8-1.2
- **Therapeutic Range for Warfarin:** 2.0-3.0 (varies depending on condition)

Interpretation:

- **High INR:** Indicates increased risk of bleeding.

- **Low INR**: Indicates risk of clotting.

Example Cases:

Case 1: Atrial Fibrillation on Warfarin

- **Presentation**: A patient with atrial fibrillation on long-term warfarin.
- **Lab Results**: INR: 3.5 (high).
- **Management**: Adjust warfarin dosage to bring INR within the therapeutic range.

Case 2: Deep Vein Thrombosis on Warfarin

- **Presentation**: A patient with a history of deep vein thrombosis.
- **Lab Results**: INR: 1.5 (low).
- **Management**: Increase warfarin dosage and recheck INR.

Case 3: Mechanical Heart Valve on Warfarin

- **Presentation**: A patient with a mechanical heart valve.
- **Lab Results**: INR: 4.0 (high).
- **Management**: Adjust warfarin dosage and monitor for signs of bleeding.

Thyroid Function Tests (TFT)

TFT are a group of blood tests used to evaluate thyroid function, which play a critical role in regulating metabolism, energy production, and overall hormonal balance in the body. TFT includes the level of thyroid stimulating hormone (TSH), free thyroxine (Free T4), and free triiodothyronine (Free T3). TSH is produced by the pituitary gland stimulating the thyroid to produce T4 and T3.

Elevated or decreased levels of TSH, along with corresponding changes in T4 and T3 levels, can indicate various thyroid disorders. For instance, high TSH and low T4 levels typically suggest hypothyroidism. Conversely, low TSH and high T4 or T3 levels may indicate hyperthyroidism.

Components of TFTs:

- **TSH (Thyroid Stimulating Hormone)**: 0.4-4.0 mIU/L
- **Free T4 (Thyroxine)**: 0.8-2.0 ng/dL
- **Free T3 (Triiodothyronine)**: 2.3-4.2 pg/mL

Interpretation:

- **High TSH, Low Free T4/Free T3**: Suggestive of hypothyroidism.
- **Low TSH, High Free T4/Free T3**: Suggestive of hyperthyroidism.

Example Cases:

Case 1: Hypothyroidism

- **Presentation**: A patient with fatigue, weight gain, and cold intolerance.
- **Lab Results**: TSH: 8.0 mIU/L (high), Free T4: 0.6 ng/dL (low).
- **Management**: Initiate levothyroxine therapy and monitor thyroid function.

Case 2: Hyperthyroidism

- **Presentation**: A patient with weight loss, palpitations, and heat intolerance.
- **Lab Results**: TSH: 0.1 mIU/L (low), Free T4: 3.0 ng/dL (high).
- **Management**: Referral to endocrinology for further evaluation and treatment.

Case 3: Subclinical Hypothyroidism

- **Presentation**: A patient with mild fatigue and normal physical examination.
- **Lab Results**: TSH: 5.5 mIU/L (slightly high), Free T4: 1.1 ng/dL (normal).
- **Management**: Monitor thyroid function and consider treatment if symptoms worsen or TSH levels rise.

High-Yield Imaging for Primary Eye Care

Computed Tomography (CT) Head and/or Orbits

CT is essentially an X-ray study, where a series of x-rays are rotated around a specified body part and computer generated images are produced. The advantage of these tomographic images compared to conventional X-rays is that they contain detailed information of a specified area in cross-section, eliminating the superimposition of images.

In a spiral or helical scan, the table moves continuously as the x-ray source and detectors rotate. This reduces the duration of the study significantly to provide quick results, especially in emergent situations. It is quickly replacing standard cerebral angiography (CTA) for detecting head trauma injuries and brain masses due to it's rapid acquisition of images.

This imaging modality is particularly effective for visualizing bone structures and acute hemorrhages, making it indispensable in the evaluation of trauma, fractures, masses, hemorrhages, and sinus conditions. CT can detect bone fractures with high sensitivity, identify acute hemorrhages through the hyperdensity of fresh blood, and assess sinus conditions by clearly imaging sinus opacification.

Generally it is good to remember CT is best for bone and blood, with MRI best for soft tissue.

Indications:

- **Brain**: Masses, traumatic or spontaneous hematomas, stroke, edema, skull fracture, calcifications, arteriovenous malformations, hydrocephalus, sinusitis, empyema.
- **Orbits**: Fractures, foreign bodies, masses, inflammation, infection.

Interpretation:

- **Brain Masses**: Well-defined or irregular masses with or without contrast enhancement.
- **Hematomas**: Hyperdense (acute) or hypodense (chronic) areas within the brain.
- **Fractures**: Discontinuities in bone structure often with surrounding soft tissue swelling.

Example Cases:

Case 1: Acute Hemorrhagic Stroke

- **Presentation**: A patient with sudden onset of severe headache, weakness on one side, and slurred speech.
- **Imaging Results**: CT shows a hyperdense area in the left hemisphere consistent with an acute hemorrhagic stroke.
- **Management**: Immediate referral to neurology for stroke management.

Case 2: Orbital Fracture

- **Presentation**: A patient with trauma to the eye and swelling.
- **Imaging Results**: CT reveals a fracture of the orbital floor with entrapment of orbital fat.
- **Management**: Referral to an oculoplastic surgeon for possible surgical intervention.

Case 3: Sinusitis

- **Presentation**: A patient with chronic headaches and nasal congestion.
- **Imaging Results**: CT shows opacification of the maxillary sinuses with mucosal thickening.
- **Management**: Referral to ENT for further evaluation and treatment.

CT Angiography (CTA)

CT Angiography (CTA) involves the injection of contrast material to visualize blood vessels, producing high-resolution images of the vascular system. This technique is foremost for detecting vascular pathologies such as aneurysms, stenosis, dissections, and arteriovenous malformations. The detailed images provided by CTA allow for the identification of aneurysms as focal out-pouchings of vessel walls, stenosis as narrowed vessel lumens, and dissections as separations of vessel wall layers.

Indications:

- **Head**: Aneurysms, stenosis, dissection, arteriovenous malformations.
- **Neck**: Carotid artery disease, vertebral artery dissection.

Interpretation:

- **Aneurysm**: Focal out-pouching of a blood vessel.
- **Stenosis**: Narrowing of the vessel lumen often with post-stenotic dilation.

Example Cases:

Case 1: Carotid Artery Stenosis

- **Presentation**: A patient with transient vision loss and a history of hypertension.
- **Imaging Results**: CTA shows 70% stenosis of the left carotid artery.
- **Management**: Referral to vascular surgery for possible carotid endarterectomy.

Case 2: Cerebral Aneurysm

- **Presentation**: A patient with a sudden severe headache.
- **Imaging Results**: CTA reveals a 5 mm aneurysm in the anterior communicating artery.
- **Management**: Referral to neurosurgery for further evaluation and possible intervention.

Case 3: Vertebral Artery Dissection

- **Presentation**: A patient with neck pain and dizziness following minor trauma.
- **Imaging Results**: CTA shows a dissection of the right vertebral artery.
- **Management**: Immediate referral to neurology for stroke prevention and management.

CT with Contrast vs CTA

CT with contrast and CTA are both advanced imaging techniques that utilize a CT scanner and intravenous contrast dye to enhance image clarity. However, they are used for different diagnostic purposes and provide distinct types of information.

CTA is specifically designed to visualize blood vessels and assess vascular conditions. It involves the injection of a contrast dye to highlight arteries and veins, making it particularly useful for diagnosing and monitoring conditions such as aneurysms, arterial blockages, and other vascular abnormalities. The enhanced imaging allows for detailed visualization of the blood vessels, facilitating precise diagnosis and aiding in the planning of interventional procedures like angioplasty or stent placement.

On the other hand, CT with contrast is a more general imaging technique that enhances the visibility of various tissues and organs, not just blood vessels. The contrast dye helps to differentiate between different types of tissues, making it useful for a broad range of diagnostic purposes, including identifying masses, infection, and other abnormalities in organs such as the liver, kidneys, and brain.

While CT with contrast provides valuable information about the anatomy and pathology of these organs, it does not offer the same level of detail regarding the vascular system as CTA.

Indications:

- **Cancer Detection and Management**: Identification and characterization of masses, assessment of size, and managing response to treatment.

- **Abdominal Pain or Trauma**: Evaluation of acute or chronic abdominal pain causes, such as appendicitis and bowel obstructions, and assessment of internal injuries following trauma, such as organ lacerations or hematomas.

Interpretation:

- **Mass or Infection**: Identification of masses, including their presence, size, location, and enhancement patterns, and detection of abscesses or cellulitis.
- **Vascular or Organ Structures**: Evaluation of vessel integrity and abnormalities such as aneurysms or dissections, and detailed visualization of abdominal and pelvic organs to detect pathology such as cysts or obstructions.

Example Cases:

Case 1: Pancreatic Cancer

- **Presentation**: A 58-year-old male presents with jaundice, weight loss, and upper abdominal pain.
- **Imaging Results**: CT with contrast reveals a hypovascular mass in the head of the

pancreas, with involvement of the bile ducts and surrounding vasculature.

- **Management**: Confirmed diagnosis of pancreatic cancer, leading to surgical planning and oncological treatment.

Case 2: Abdominal Aortic Aneurysm (AAA) with Dissection

- **Presentation**: A 72-year-old female with severe back pain and hypotension, with a history of hypertension and smoking.
- **Imaging Results**: CT with contrast shows a large abdominal aortic aneurysm with an intimal flap and dissection extending into the iliac arteries.
- **Management**: Immediate surgical intervention to repair the aneurysm and prevent rupture.

Case 3: Acute Appendicitis

- **Presentation**: A 23-year-old female with right lower quadrant abdominal pain, fever, and elevated white blood cell count.
- **Imaging Results**: CT with contrast shows an enlarged, inflamed appendix with surrounding fat stranding and an appendicolith.
- **Management**: Confirmed diagnosis of acute appendicitis, leading to prompt surgical consultation and appendectomy.

Magnetic Resonance Imaging (MRI) Brain and/or Orbits

MRI uses powerful magnets and radio waves to generate detailed images of soft tissues, making it the preferred method for evaluating the brain and orbits. A major advantage is the ability to produce high-quality images with superior contrast without using ionizing radiation. The ability to evaluate structural integrity with respect to soft tissue lends the MRI for imaging the neural axis, abdominopelvic region, as well as cardio-thoracic imaging.

The magnet generates images based on specific and unique magnetic properties of tissues driven by spin properties of hydrogen molecules. This also makes the MRI especially useful to evaluate "high radiation risk" individuals like pregnant women and children.

MRI is particularly high-yield for detecting malignancies, which appear as masses, and identifying multiple sclerosis or demyelinating plaques as hyperintense lesions on T2-weighted images. It is also essential for diagnosing and managing conditions including stroke, meningitis, encephalitis, optic neuritis, inflammatory bowel disease, and others.

Whether or not to use a contrast agent, usually gadolinium based contrast, depends on the nature of the disease/condition suspected for which you are ordering the imaging. Most acute events such as headache, potential stroke, transient ischemic attack suspects, or head trauma with a potential brain bleed vs concussion, do not require a contrast MRI.

Other conditions including suspicion of a mass or space occupying lesion, a potential inflammatory or infectious source, seizure disorders, demyelinating disease like MS, and others do require the use of a contrast agent to differentiate diseased tissue from normal tissue.

Indications:

- **Brain**: masses, multiple sclerosis, stroke, infection, demyelinating disease.
- **Orbits**: Optic neuritis, masses, inflammation, vascular anomalies.

Interpretation:

- **Masses**: With or without contrast enhancement, possibly causing displacement of adjacent structures.
- **Multiple Sclerosis**: Lesions in the white matter, often periventricular, enhancing with contrast during active inflammation.

Example Cases:

Case 1: Multiple Sclerosis

- **Presentation**: A patient with intermittent vision loss and tingling in the extremities.
- **Imaging Results**: MRI shows multiple hyperintense lesions in the periventricular white matter.
- **Management**: Referral to neurology for further evaluation and disease-modifying therapy.

Case 2: Optic Neuritis

- **Presentation**: A patient with acute vision loss and pain on eye movement.
- **Imaging Results**: MRI shows enhancement of the optic nerve with contrast.
- **Management**: Referral to neurology for evaluation of possible multiple sclerosis and initiation of corticosteroids.

Case 3: Brain Mass

- **Presentation**: A patient with persistent headaches and visual field defects.
- **Imaging Results**: MRI reveals a contrast-enhancing mass in the occipital lobe.
- **Management**: Referral to neurosurgery for biopsy and treatment planning.

Magnetic Resonance Angiography (MRA)

Magnetic Resonance Angiography (MRA) is a specialized MRI technique focused on visualizing vasculature. This technique is valuable for detecting intracranial aneurysms, arteriovenous malformations, and assessing stenosis in arteries, providing clear images of blood flow and vessel structure.

MRA should be considered in patients with diminished renal function and preferred over CTA by understanding MRA utilizing *Time of Flight* (TOF) does not require contrast (usually gadolinium). It is a multidimensional 2D or 3D technique mapping the imaged vessels, then "subtracting" the bony structures and brain parenchyma. It uses flow-related enhancement properties during image acquisition rather than relying on contrast agents.

Indications:

- **Brain**: Aneurysms, arteriovenous malformations, stenosis.
- **Neck**: Carotid artery disease, vertebral artery dissection.

Interpretation:

- **Aneurysms**: Focal dilatations of blood vessels, often detected without the need for contrast.

- **Stenosis**: Narrowing of vessel lumen visible as a reduced flow signal on TOF MRA.

Example Cases:

Case 1: Intracranial Aneurysm

- **Presentation**: A patient with sudden onset of a severe headache.
- **Imaging Results**: MRA reveals a 6 mm aneurysm in the middle cerebral artery.
- **Management**: Referral to neurosurgery for further evaluation and potential intervention.

Case 2: Carotid Artery Stenosis

- **Presentation**: A patient with transient ischemic attacks.
- **Imaging Results**: MRA shows significant stenosis of the right internal carotid artery.
- **Management**: Referral to vascular surgery for further evaluation and possible intervention.

Case 3: Arteriovenous Malformation

- **Presentation**: A patient with seizures and headaches.
- **Imaging Results**: MRA reveals a complex arteriovenous malformation in the left temporal lobe.

- **Management**: Referral to neurosurgery for evaluation and treatment planning.

Magnetic Resonance Venography (MRV)

MRV is a specialized imaging technique using magnetic resonance imaging (MRI) technology to visualize the venous system, particularly those in the brain and neck. Unlike traditional MRI which focuses on tissues and organs, MRV specifically highlights venous structures, making it an invaluable tool for diagnosing and managing related conditions. The process involves the use of a contrast agent (usually gadolinium) which is injected into the bloodstream, enhancing the visibility of venous circulation. This allows for detailed images which can reveal abnormalities such as deep venous thrombosis (DVT), venous malformations, and other vasculopathies. It is also employed to evaluate venous anatomy before various surgical procedures.

The non-invasive nature of MRV, combined with its ability to provide high-resolution images without the use of ionizing radiation, makes it a preferred method for detailed venous assessment ensuring accurate diagnosis and aiding in effective management.

MRV is particularly useful in diagnosing dural venous sinus thrombosis (DVST). The dural venous sinuses can also be evaluated with *time of flight* (TOF) MRV, which does not require the use of contrast agents. For example, with suspected idiopathic intracranial hypertension (IIH)/pseudotumor patients, dural venous sinus thrombosis is present in more than 90% of cases.

Indications:

- **Cerebral Venous Thrombosis**: Suspected venous sinus thrombosis.
- **Venous Malformations**: Evaluation of abnormal venous structures.

Interpretation:

- **Venous Thrombosis**: Absence of flow signal in the venous sinuses or cerebral veins.
- **Venous Malformations**: Abnormal or dilated venous structures, often with irregular flow patterns.

Example Cases:

Case 1: Cerebral Venous Thrombosis

- **Presentation**: A patient with severe headache, nausea, and papilledema.
- **Imaging Results**: MRV shows absence of flow in the superior sagittal sinus, consistent with venous thrombosis.
- **Management**: Immediate referral to neurology for anticoagulation therapy and further management.

Case 2: Idiopathic Intracranial Hypertension

- **Presentation**: A patient with chronic headaches and visual disturbances.
- **Imaging Results**: MRV reveals stenosis of the transverse sinuses, supporting a diagnosis of increased intracranial pressure.
- **Management**: Referral to neurology for further evaluation and management, including possible lumbar puncture and medication to reduce intracranial pressure.

Case 3: Venous Angioma

- **Presentation**: A patient with a history of seizures and headaches.
- **Imaging Results**: MRV shows a cluster of dilated veins in the left parietal region, consistent with a venous angioma.
- **Management**: Referral to neurosurgery for further evaluation and discussion of potential treatment options.

FIESTA Protocol MRI

The FIESTA (Fast Imaging Employing Steady-state Acquisition) protocol is a specialized non-contrast MRI technique renowned for its ability to produce high-resolution images with excellent tissue contrast.

This technique leverages the inherent differences in the magnetic properties of various tissues, making it particularly effective for visualizing fine anatomic details in structures such as the brain, inner ear, cranial nerves, and cerebrospinal fluid spaces. Its applications extend to cardiac imaging and the great vessels, as well as musculoskeletal imaging for joints and cartilage.

It is superior for visualizing cranial nerve lesions especially along the posterior fossa, including neuronal compression, masses, as well as detailing brainstem abnormalities. It is particularly useful for conditions like trigeminal neuralgia and vestibular schwannoma.

Another advantage of the FIESTA protocol is its rapid image acquisition, which is highly beneficial in clinical settings where time is of the essence. Additionally, the elimination of gadolinium-based contrast agents makes it a safer option for patients with contraindications to contrast media, such as those with renal impairment.

Consider this protocol when targeting a potential III, IV, or VI nerve palsy.

Indications:

- **Cranial Nerve Evaluation**: Trigeminal neuralgia, vestibular schwannoma.
- **Detailed Brain Imaging**: Evaluation of brainstem and posterior fossa structures.

Interpretation:

- **Cranial Nerve Lesions**: High-resolution images allow for the detection of nerve compression or masses.
- **Brainstem Abnormalities**: Clear visualization of brainstem structures for detailed assessment.

Example Cases:

Case 1: Trigeminal Neuralgia

- **Presentation**: A patient with severe facial pain.
- **Imaging Results**: FIESTA MRI shows vascular compression of the trigeminal nerve.
- **Management**: Referral to neurosurgery for potential microvascular decompression.

Case 2: Vestibular Schwannoma

- **Presentation**: A patient with hearing loss and tinnitus.
- **Imaging Results**: FIESTA MRI reveals a mass on the vestibulocochlear nerve.
- **Management**: Referral to neurosurgery or otolaryngology for further evaluation and management.

Case 3: Brainstem Glioma

- **Presentation**: A patient with progressive difficulty swallowing and speech changes.
- **Imaging Results**: FIESTA MRI shows an infiltrative lesion in the brainstem.
- **Management**: Referral to oncology for further evaluation and treatment planning.

Echocardiogram (Echo)

Echo is a non-invasive imaging technique which utilizes ultrasound to create detailed images of the heart. This procedure provides valuable information regarding cardiac function and blood flow by assessing cardiac musculature, valves, and chambers. By placing a transducer on the patient's chest, sound waves are directed towards the heart, and the returning echoes are captured to form real-time images on a monitor.

In addition to standard transthoracic echocardiogram (TTE), another advanced form of echocardiography is the transesophageal echocardiogram (TEE). While under sedation, TEE involves passing a specialized transducer down the patient's esophagus, which is posterior and in close proximity to the heart. This approach provides clearer and more detailed images of the heart's structures, especially the posterior regions and valves which can be difficult to visualize with TTE.

TEE is particularly useful in diagnosing conditions such as endocarditis, atrial fibrillation, and detecting blood clots or assessing valve function post-surgery. Although more invasive, TEE is highly valuable for its enhanced imaging capabilities and is often used when precise cardiac evaluation is necessary.

Both TTE and TEE are safe, effective, and do not involve radiation making them essential tools in cardiac diagnostics.

Indications:

- **Structural Abnormalities**: Valvular heart disease, cardiomyopathy.
- **Functional Assessment**: Ejection fraction, cardiac output.

Interpretation:

- **Valvular Disease**: Abnormal valve structure or function such as stenosis or regurgitation.
- **Cardiomyopathy**: Enlarged heart chambers, reduced ejection fraction.

Example Cases:

Case 1: Mitral Valve Prolapse

- **Presentation**: A patient with palpitations and chest discomfort.
- **Imaging Results**: Echo shows prolapse of the mitral valve leaflets with mild regurgitation.

- **Management**: Monitoring and symptomatic treatment, referral to cardiology if symptoms worsen.

Case 2: Dilated Cardiomyopathy

- **Presentation**: A patient with shortness of breath and fatigue.
- **Imaging Results**: Echo reveals dilated left ventricle with reduced ejection fraction.
- **Management**: Referral to cardiology for further evaluation and management, including possible medications and lifestyle modifications.

Case 3: Aortic Stenosis

- **Presentation**: An elderly patient with exertional dyspnea and a heart murmur.
- **Imaging Results**: Echo shows thickened aortic valve leaflets with significant stenosis and a high transvalvular gradient.
- **Management**: Referral to cardiology for evaluation and potential aortic valve replacement.

Carotid Duplex or Doppler Ultrasound

Carotid duplex ultrasound combines traditional ultrasound with doppler ultrasound to evaluate blood flow in the carotid arteries. This technique is superior for assessing carotid artery disease, stroke risk, and evaluating the patency of carotid arteries. Carotid duplex measures blood flow velocity to detect stenosis or occlusion, providing important information regarding stroke risk assessment and prevention.

Indications:

- **Carotid Artery Disease**: Stenosis, occlusion.
- **Stroke/TIA Evaluation**: Assessment of carotid artery patency.

Interpretation:

- **Stenosis**: Narrowing of the carotid artery indicated by increased blood flow velocity.
- **Occlusion**: Complete blockage of the carotid artery indicated by absence of blood flow.

Example Cases:

Case 1: Carotid Artery Stenosis

- **Presentation**: A patient with transient ischemic attacks.
- **Imaging Results**: Carotid duplex shows 70% stenosis of the left internal carotid artery.
- **Management**: Referral to vascular surgery for potential carotid endarterectomy.

Case 2: Carotid Artery Occlusion

- **Presentation**: A patient with sudden onset of weakness on one side.
- **Imaging Results**: Carotid duplex reveals complete occlusion of the right internal carotid artery.
- **Management**: Referral to neurology for stroke management.

Case 3: Carotid Plaque

- **Presentation**: A patient with no symptoms but with a family history of stroke.
- **Imaging Results**: Carotid duplex shows atherosclerotic plaque with mild stenosis.
- **Management**: Lifestyle modifications and medical management to prevent progression.

Electrodiagnostic Investigations

Electrocardiogram (ECG/EKG)

An ECG records the heart's electrical activity to assess rhythm, rate, and conduction pathways. By placing electrodes on the skin at specific anatomical locations, chest, arms, and legs, the ECG captures electrical impulses generated by the depolarization and repolarization of the cardiac musculature. These impulses are then translated into characteristic waveforms (P wave, QRS complex, T wave) displayed on a monitor or printed on paper, each corresponding to different phases of the cardiac cycle.

ECG's are indispensable in diagnosing and monitoring a variety of cardiac conditions. It provides detailed insights into arrhythmias such as atrial fibrillation, ventricular tachycardia, and heart blocks, helping to pinpoint abnormalities in the heart's electrical conduction system.

ECG's are critical in acute settings for detecting myocardial ischemia and infarction, indicated by changes such as ST-segment elevation or depression, T wave inversion, and the presence of pathological Q waves. It also aids in assessing electrolyte disturbances such as hyperkalemia, hypokalemia, and others, as well as the effects of cardiotoxic drugs.

Indications:

- **Cardiac Symptoms**: Palpitations, chest pain, syncope.
- **Preoperative Evaluation**: Assessment before non-cardiac surgery.

Interpretation:

- **Myocardial Infarction**: ST-segment elevation, pathological Q waves.
- **Arrhythmias**: Abnormal heart rhythms such as atrial fibrillation or ventricular tachycardia.

Example Cases:

Case 1: Myocardial Infarction

- **Presentation**: A patient with acute chest pain radiating to the left arm.
- **Imaging Results**: ECG shows ST-segment elevation in leads II, III, and aVF.
- **Management**: Immediate referral to emergency department for intervention.

Case 2: Atrial Fibrillation

- **Presentation**: A patient with palpitations and shortness of breath.
- **Imaging Results**: ECG reveals irregularly irregular rhythm with no distinct P waves.
- **Management**: Referral to cardiology for rate control and anticoagulation management.

Case 3: Ventricular Tachycardia

- **Presentation**: A patient with dizziness and syncope.
- **Imaging Results**: ECG shows wide QRS complex tachycardia.
- **Management**: Immediate referral to emergency department for stabilization and treatment.

Electroencephalogram (EEG)

EEG is a non-invasive diagnostic modality measuring electrical activity of the brain. By placing electrodes on the scalp, the EEG captures spontaneous electrical activity generated by neuronal firing and records it as waveforms. These waveforms represent different brain wave patterns, such as alpha, beta, delta, and theta waves, which correspond to various states of brain activity, from wakefulness to deep sleep.

EEG's are essential for diagnosing and managing neurologic conditions, particularly seizure disorders, for which abnormal electrical discharges in the brain are detected as epileptiform activity. It is also utilized to assess brain function in patients with disorders such as encephalopathy, sleep disorders, and brain death.

In clinical practice, EEG's can help identify the location and extent of brain abnormalities, guide treatment decisions, and monitor the effectiveness of interventions. The procedure is safe, painless, and can be performed in both inpatient and outpatient settings, making it a versatile tool in neurologic diagnostics.

Indications:

- **Seizure Disorders:** Diagnosis and monitoring.
- **Encephalopathy:** Evaluation of altered mental status.
- **Sleep Disorders:** Assessment of sleep patterns and disturbances.

Interpretation:

- **Seizures:** Abnormal electrical discharges such as spikes and sharp waves.
- **Encephalopathy:** Diffuse slowing of background activity.

Example Cases:

Case 1: Epilepsy

- **Presentation:** A patient with recurrent unprovoked seizures.
- **Imaging Results:** EEG shows generalized spike-and-wave discharges.
- **Management:** Referral to neurology for anticonvulsant therapy and further evaluation.

Case 2: Encephalopathy

- **Presentation:** A patient with confusion and altered mental status.
- **Imaging Results:** EEG reveals diffuse slowing of background activity.
- **Management:** Evaluation for underlying cause and appropriate treatment

Case 3: Sleep Apnea

- **Presentation:** A patient with excessive daytime sleepiness and snoring.
- **Imaging Results:** EEG during a sleep study shows frequent arousals associated with apneic episodes.
- **Management:** Referral to a sleep specialist for CPAP therapy and lifestyle modifications.

Visual Evoked Potentials (VEP)

VEP is a safe and non-invasive diagnostic procedure utilized to evaluate functional integrity of the visual pathway, from retina to the occipital cortex. It measures the brain's electrical response to visual stimuli providing valuable information about the entire visual system.

Electrodes are strategically placed on the scalp over the occipital region and the patient is asked to focus on specific visual stimuli, such as a checkerboard pattern or flashing lights presented on a monitor. The electrical activity generated by the visual cortex in response to these stimuli is recorded and analyzed.

VEP is particularly valuable in diagnosing and managing neurologic conditions affecting the optic nerve. This includes optic neuritis in multiple sclerosis and other optic neuropathies. The procedure detects delays or abnormalities in the transmission of visual signals, which can be indicative of pathology.

VEP is also instrumental in evaluating visual function in patients with unexplained vision loss, confirming a diagnosis of optic neuropathy and assessing the visual system pre- and post-operatively for surgical interventions like optic nerve decompression.

By measuring latency and amplitude of visual responses, VEP provides detailed information on conduction velocity and functional status of the visual pathway, making it an essential tool in both clinical practice and research settings.

Indications:

- **Optic Nerve Disorders**: Diagnosis and monitoring.
- **Unexplained Visual Loss**: Assessment of visual function.
- **Head Injuries**: Evaluation of visual pathway integrity.

Interpretation:

- **Normal VEP**: Well-defined waves, with the P100 wave being the most prominent and reliable marker.
- **Abnormal VEP**: Delayed latency or reduced amplitude of the P100 wave, indicating dysfunction in the visual pathway.

Example Cases:

Case 1: Multiple Sclerosis

- **Presentation**: A 30-year-old female presents with sudden blurred vision in her right eye.
- **Imaging Results**: VEP shows delayed P100 latency in the affected eye compared to the normal eye.
- **Management**: Suggestive of demyelination of

the optic nerve, consistent with multiple
sclerosis.

Case 2: Optic Neuritis

- **Presentation**: A 25-year-old male reports
  pain and temporary vision loss in his left eye.
- **Imaging Results**: VEP shows prolonged
  P100 latency in the left eye with normal
  findings in the right eye.
- **Management**: Indicative of optic neuritis,
  likely due to inflammation or infection
  affecting the optic nerve.

Case 3: Head Injury

- **Presentation**: A 40-year-old male with a
  history of traumatic brain injury presents with
  visual disturbances.
- **Imaging Results**: VEP shows reduced
  amplitude and delayed P100 latency in both
  eyes.
- **Management**: Suggests damage to the visual
  pathways possibly due to the trauma,
  requiring further neurological evaluation.

Electroretinogram (ERG)

ERG is a non-invasive diagnostic modality which
measures electrical responses of the retina,
specifically photoreceptors (rods and cones) and

inner retinal cells (bipolar and ganglion cells), to light stimuli.

A patient is typically seated in a darkened room and allowed time to visually adapt. Electrodes are placed on the cornea using a contact lens and on the skin around the eye to record electrical activity. The individual is then exposed to various light stimuli, and the resulting electrical responses are recorded.

ERG is key for diagnosing and managing a variety of retinal disorders, including retinitis pigmentosa (RP) and cone-rod dystrophies. It helps in assessing the functional state of the retina, when structural assessments such as ophthalmoscopy or optical coherence tomography (OCT) might not provide sufficient information. By analyzing different components of the ERG waveform, it can be determined which specific layers or types of cells in the retina are affected.

The ERG is also valuable in evaluating unexplained vision loss and can be used pre- and post-operatively to assess retinal function in patients undergoing procedures such as retinal detachment surgery.

Indications:

- **Inherited Retinal Disorders**: Diagnosis and management.
- **Unexplained Vision Loss**: Evaluation of retinal function.

- **Retinal Toxicity**: Assessment due to medications or substances.

Interpretation:

- **Normal ERG**: Well-defined a-waves and b-waves representing photoreceptor and bipolar cell activity.
- **Abnormal ERG**: Reduced amplitude or absent waves, indicating retinal dysfunction.

Example Cases:

Case 1: Retinitis Pigmentosa

- **Presentation**: A 20-year-old male presents with progressive night blindness and peripheral vision loss.
- **Imaging Results**: ERG shows markedly reduced rod responses with diminished a- and b-waves under scotopic (dark-adapted) conditions.
- **Management**: Consistent with rod photoreceptor degeneration, indicative of retinitis pigmentosa.

Case 2: Diabetic Retinopathy

- **Presentation**: A 50-year-old female with a history of diabetes complains of blurred vision and floaters.

- **Imaging Results**: ERG shows reduced amplitude of both a- and b-waves, indicating widespread retinal dysfunction.
- **Management**: Suggestive of retinal damage due to diabetic retinopathy, requiring further management and treatment.

Case 3: Drug Toxicity

- **Presentation**: A 35-year-old male on long-term hydroxychloroquine therapy for lupus reports vision changes.
- **Imaging Results**: ERG shows decreased cone responses with reduced photopic (light-adapted) b-wave amplitudes.
- **Management**: Indicative of cone dysfunction likely due to drug toxicity, necessitating reassessment of the medication regimen.

Writing The Scripts

Steps for Writing an Order:

Imaging

When preparing a written order for imaging, echocardiogram, and others, you must first be credentialed and participate in the patient's medical insurance to be authorized. This ensures your patient will be received at the imaging center or hospital without incident.

Written Script:

1. **Write Specific Studies:** Names and current CPT codes.
2. **Write Working Diagnosis or Differentials**: Use current ICD-10 codes.
3. **Authorization**: Your staff should contact the insurance carrier and imaging center or hospital for a verbal authorization. Some

insurance carriers provide online authorization to streamline the process.

4. **Fax Script**: Fax your written script to both the insurance carrier and the imaging center.

Example of a script for an MRI Brain with contrast:

- **Investigation**: MRI Brain with contrast
- **CPT Code**: 70553
- **Working Diagnosis**: Optic Neuritis
- **ICD-10 Code**: H46.9

Instructions for Patients:

Inform patients the authorization might take up to 48 hours. Individuals with non-urgent scenarios can be sent home and contacted when the authorization is complete. Urgent imaging can be arranged via coordinating stat authorization with a free-standing center, or in the ED by calling ahead and communicating your rationale with appropriate staff.

Labs

1. **No Prior Authorization Needed**: You are free to order laboratory investigations if credentialed with the patient's medical insurance.
2. **Written Script Requirements**: Include all labs you are requesting. CPT codes are not required. However, include on the written

script ICD-10 diagnostic codes supporting your diagnosis or differentials.

3. **Fasting Instructions**: Inform the patient if fasting is required (e.g., lipid profile, glucose).

Example of a Script for a CMP:

- **Investigation**: Comprehensive Metabolic Profile (CMP)
- **Working Diagnosis**: Uncontrolled Type II Diabetes Mellitus
- **ICD-10 Code**: E11.65
- **Fasting Required**: Yes

Results:

Lab and imaging results are automatically sent allowing you to better manage your patient. With regard to imaging such as MRI or CT, requesting disc copies for your review is not necessary. You will receive the radiology read and/or lab report. Your role is to understand the report and its language to support or refute your working diagnosis. In your clinical judgement, you may also occasionally disagree with the findings or suspect further investigations are necessary.

Logistics

True primary eye care includes and incorporates comprehensive medical management, including the utilization of outside labs and imaging. As an optometrist, you fill a significant and glaring gap bridging general medicine and surgical ophthalmology. Your effective communication and collaboration with specialists are key to providing proper care.

When it comes to interpreting and managing labs or imaging results, it's important to recognize the distinction between interpretation and management. The interpretation and report produced by other specialists does not equate to you managing your patient. Your responsibility is to utilize reports to support or refute your working diagnosis, ensuring your patient's clinical picture is managed and understood. Also keep in mind, laboratory results can change daily.

Be aware radiology reads are subjective analyses by radiologists, and there is always the potential for human error and technological glitches. It's essential to consider these factors as well when evaluating diagnostic reports.

In terms of communication, you will frequently engage with various medical specialties. As examples, you might communicate with cardiologists regarding a person with stroke-like symptoms, TIA's, sudden visual field defects, or acute diplopia. Obstetricians/gynecologists consulted for individuals with PCOS and fluctuating vision related to glucose levels. Endocrinologists are involved for cases of prolactinomas and potential field loss. Rheumatologists are important for managing SLE/lupus patients presenting with recurrent uveitis. Neurologists are highly pertinent in your practice for conditions like multiple sclerosis or optic neuritis.

To be effective, it's essential to communicate your impressions and recommendations directly. Make appropriate referrals and share your findings comprehensively. Automatically include yourself on the medical team, collaborating with other specialists to ensure your patients receive the best possible care. By doing so, you help create a cohesive and thorough approach to management.

Conclusion

In primary medical eye care, which is optometry, the integration of labs and imaging diagnostics is not merely an enhancement but a necessity for providing comprehensive care. It is imperative to expand your daily scope of practice to include these essential diagnostic tools, ensuring you deliver the highest standard of care to your patients.

This book has aimed to equip you with some foundational knowledge required to help effectively order and utilize labs and imaging in your daily practice. By becoming comfortable in comprehensive management, you are better positioned to make informed decisions, provide timely interventions, and ultimately improve patient outcomes. The examples given are designed to serve as a very basic practical reference, reinforcing your confidence in managing diverse clinical scenarios.

Remember, the journey to mastering lab and imaging diagnostics is continuous. It involves a commitment to ongoing education, collaboration with other healthcare professionals, and an empathetic priority to take responsibility for your patients problem. Your role is foremost in bridging the gap between general medicine and specialized surgical ophthalmic care. By embracing expanded responsibility, you not only enhance your clinical capabilities but also contribute to the advancement and recognition of optometry within the medical community.

Stay curious, stay diligent, and continue to seek out new knowledge and skills. Primary medical eye care presents endless opportunities for growth and improvement. Strive to provide holistic patient-centered care that meets the highest standards.

Thank you for your dedication to the specialty of optometry and for your commitment to the well-being of your patients.

John R. Martinelli
June 30, 2024

Resources

Labs

Lab Tests Online (https://labtestsonline.org/)

A resource providing detailed information on various laboratory tests, including indications, procedures, and interpretation of results.

ARUP Consult (https://arupconsult.com/)

An online resource offering expert advice on test selection and interpretation to assist clinicians in making informed decisions about laboratory testing.

LabCorp (https://www.labcorp.com/)

Provides a wide range of laboratory testing services and resources for clinicians, including test directories and patient information.

Quest Diagnostics (https://www.questdiagnostics.com/)

Offers comprehensive diagnostic testing services and resources, including test ordering guides, patient preparation instructions, and result interpretation support.

Mayo Clinic Laboratories (https://www. mayocliniclabs.com/)

A comprehensive resource offering clinical laboratory testing, test catalogs, and educational materials to assist healthcare providers in test selection and interpretation.

Imaging

Radiology (https://pubs.rsna.org/journal/radiology) Tools & Resources

American College of Radiology (https://pubs.rsna. org/journal/radiology) (ACR) **Appropriateness Criteria** (https://www.acr.org/Clinical-Resources/ACR-Appropriateness-Criteria)

Guidelines that assist clinicians in making appropriate imaging decisions, ensuring the best possible patient care.

Radiopaedia (https://radiopaedia.org/)

An extensive resource for radiology, offering educational articles, case studies, and a rich image database for various imaging modalities.

Radiology (https://pubs.rsna.org/journal/radiology) Assistant (https://radiologyassistant.nl/)

An educational resource offering detailed tutorials and case studies on interpreting radiological images.

Diagnostic Imaging (https://www. diagnosticimaging.com/)

A comprehensive resource offering news, education, and case studies related to diagnostic imaging.

Diagnostic ICD10 & Procedural CPT Reference

ICD10 Consult App (https://www.icd10data.com/)

Provides comprehensive access to ICD-10 codes, helping you accurately code diagnoses and facilitate proper billing.

CPT Codes PDF: CMS Image (https://www.cms.gov/ medicare/coding/icd10)

A downloadable PDF providing a detailed list of radiology CPT codes to facilitate accurate billing and coding for imaging procedures.

Prescribing Tools

E-Scribe App: iPrescribe (https://www.drfirst.com/ eprescribing/iprescribe/)

A digital tool providing a streamlined process for

electronic prescriptions, improving efficiency and accuracy in medication management.

Epocrates (https://www.epocrates.com/)

An app that offers drug information, including dosing, interactions, and side effects, to help healthcare providers prescribe medications safely.

Medscape (https://www.medscape.com/) **Drug Interaction Checker** (https://reference.medscape. com/drug-interactionchecker)

An online tool that helps healthcare providers check for potential drug interactions to ensure patient safety.

Continuing Medical Education

Medscape (https://www.medscape.com/)

Offers a wide range of continuing medical education (CME) courses, articles, and news updates to help medical professionals stay current in their field.

UpToDate (https://www.uptodate.com/)

An evidence-based clinical resource that provides continuously updated information on a wide range of medical topics, helping clinicians make informed decisions.

CME Webinars and Conferences

Various medical organizations provide webinars and conferences that offer CME credits. These events cover the latest advancements in medical research, technologies, and clinical practices.

Coursera (https://www.coursera.org/)

Offers online courses in various medical and health-related fields, many of which provide CME credits.

Patient Education

Mayo Clinic Patient Education (https://www.mayoclinic.org/patient-education)

Offers comprehensive resources and guides on various health conditions, treatments, and preventive care to help patients understand and manage their health.

WebMD (https://www.webmd.com/)

Provides health information, tools for managing your health, and support to those who seek information. It covers a broad spectrum of health topics and is a reliable source for patient education.

MedlinePlus (https://medlineplus.gov/)

A service of the National Library of Medicine (NLM) providing information about diseases, conditions, and wellness issues in language that is easy to understand.

KidsHealth (https://kidshealth.org/)

Offers health information for parents, kids, and teens, providing reliable information about growth, development, and health issues.

Research Databases

PubMed (https://pubmed.ncbi.nlm.nih.gov/)

A free resource developed by the National Center for Biotechnology Information (NCBI) that includes over 30 million citations for biomedical literature from MEDLINE, life science journals, and online books.

Cochrane Library (https://www.cochranelibrary.com/)

A collection of high-quality, independent evidence to inform healthcare decision-making. It includes reliable and up-to-date information from Cochrane Reviews.

Google Scholar (https://scholar.google.com/)

A freely accessible web search engine that indexes the full text or metadata of scholarly literature across an array of publishing formats and disciplines.

ResearchGate (https://www.researchgate.net/)

A professional network for scientists and researchers to share papers, ask and answer questions, and find collaborators.

ClinicalTrials.gov (https://clinicaltrials.gov/)

A database of privately and publicly funded clinical studies conducted around the world, providing information on the purpose, eligibility, locations, and contacts of studies.

Professional Organizations

American Medical Association (AMA) (https://www.ama-assn.org/)

The AMA is an organization of physicians dedicated to promoting the art and science of medicine and the betterment of public health.

Radiological Society of North America (RSNA) (https://www.rsna.org/)

An international society of radiologists, medical physicists, and other medical professionals that provides educational resources, research funding, and annual meetings to advance the practice of radiology.

American College of Physicians (ACP) (https://www.acponline.org/)

A professional organization for internal medicine physicians (internists). The ACP provides professional development resources, guidelines, and advocacy for internists.

American Board of Medical Specialties (ABMS) (https://www.abms.org/)

A non-profit organization overseeing physician certification in the United States, providing information on board certification and professional standards.

American Academy of Pediatrics (AAP) (https://www.aap.org/)

An organization of pediatricians dedicated to the health, safety, and well-being of infants, children, adolescents, and young adults.

American College of Surgeons (ACS) (https://www.facs.org/)

A scientific and educational association of surgeons aimed at improving the quality of care for surgical patients by setting high standards for surgical education and practice.

American Academy of Optometry (AAO) (https://www.aaopt.org/)

An organization dedicated to the advancement of optometric practice and research, providing education and resources to optometrists.

American Optometric Association (AOA) (https://www.aoa.org/)

A professional association representing doctors of optometry, offering resources for clinical practice, professional development, and advocacy.

American Academy of Ophthalmology (https://www.aaojournal.org/) (AAO) (https://www.aao.org/)

The largest national membership association of eye physicians and surgeons, dedicated to advancing the lifelong learning and professional interests of ophthalmologists.

Medical Journals

The New England Journal of Medicine (NEJM) (https://www.nejm.org/)

A leading medical journal that publishes peer-reviewed research and review articles in all areas of medicine.

The Lancet (https://www.thelancet.com/)

One of the world's oldest and best-known general medical journals, publishing high-quality research articles.

Journal of the American Medical Association (JAMA) (https://jamanetwork.com/journals/jama)

A peer-reviewed medical journal published by the American Medical Association, covering all aspects of the medical field.

BMJ (British Medical Journal) (https://www.bmj.com/)

A weekly peer-reviewed medical journal that provides a wide range of research articles and reviews.

Radiology (https://pubs.rsna.org/journal/radiology)

The official journal of the Radiological Society of North America (RSNA) (https://www.rsna.org/), providing peer-reviewed articles on clinical radiology and related disciplines.

Journal of Clinical Oncology (JCO) (https://ascopubs.org/journal/jco)

A leading oncology journal providing clinical research articles on the treatment of cancer.

Nature Medicine (https://www.nature.com/nm/)

A highly regarded journal publishing original research articles across all areas of medicine.

Annals of Internal Medicine (https://www.acpjournals.org/journal/aim)

A premier internal medicine journal publishing research, reviews, guidelines, and commentary relevant to clinical practice and health policy.

Ophthalmology (https://www.aaojournal.org/)

The official journal of the American Academy of Ophthalmology (https://www.aaojournal.org/), publishing peer-reviewed articles on all aspects of eye care.

Journal of Cataract and Refractive Surgery (https://www.jcrsjournal.org/)

A leading journal focused on clinical and research developments in cataract and refractive surgery.

Optometry and Vision Science (https://journals.lww.com/optvissci/pages/default.aspx)

The official journal of the American Academy of Optometry, providing peer-reviewed research and clinical articles on optometry and vision science.

Investigative Ophthalmology (https://www.aaojournal.org/) & Visual Science (IOVS)

A peer-reviewed journal publishing research on clinical and laboratory investigations related to ophthalmology and vision science.

Test Your Knowledge

1. What are the clinical implications of a persistently high ESR in a patient with recurrent uveitis, and how should an optometrist proceed with the management?

a) Suggests chronic infection; prescribe antibiotics.

b) Indicates inflammatory or autoimmune etiology; refer to rheumatology.

c) Reflects dehydration; recommend increased fluid intake.

d) Suggests liver dysfunction; order liver function tests.

2. When encountering a patient with sudden vision loss and a WBC count of 50,000 cells/mcL with blasts, what immediate steps should be taken?

a) Prescribe antibiotics for infection.

b) Refer urgently to hematology/oncology for suspected acute leukemia.

c) Monitor and recheck WBC in one week.

d) Recommend rest and hydration.

3. How can an optometrist differentiate between anemia due to chronic disease and iron deficiency anemia using CBC results?

a) Evaluate platelet counts.

b) Compare hemoglobin levels.

c) Assess mean corpuscular volume (MCV) and red cell distribution width (RDW).

d) Check white blood cell differential.

4. What are the indications for ordering a CT Angiography (CTA) in a patient with visual field defects and suspected stroke?

a) Assessing for carotid artery stenosis or intracranial aneurysms.

b) Evaluating optic nerve swelling.

c) Checking for sinus infection.

d) Diagnosing retinal detachment.

5. In a patient with suspected multiple sclerosis presenting with optic neuritis, what imaging modality and findings would support this diagnosis?

a) CT scan showing brain atrophy.

b) MRI showing periventricular white matter lesions.

c) Ultrasound showing retinal detachment.

d) X-ray showing calcifications.

6. **What is the significance of a high CRP level in conjunction with normal ESR in a patient with acute vision changes?**

a) Indicates bacterial infection; prescribe antibiotics.

b) Suggests a non-specific inflammatory response; further evaluation needed.

c) Reflects chronic inflammation; refer to rheumatology.

d) Points to viral infection; monitor and provide supportive care.

7. **How does the presence of anti-nuclear antibodies (ANA) with a speckled pattern assist in the differential diagnosis of systemic lupus erythematosus (SLE) and Sjögren's syndrome?**

a) ANA with a speckled pattern is more specific for SLE.

b) ANA with a speckled pattern is indicative of Sjögren's syndrome.

c) Speckled pattern alone cannot differentiate; clinical correlation is essential.

d) Speckled pattern rules out SLE.

8. What are the potential complications of a patient with poorly controlled diabetes, high fasting blood glucose, and elevated HbA1c presenting with fluctuating vision?

a) Risk of diabetic retinopathy and macular edema.

b) Increased likelihood of optic neuritis.

c) High risk of retinal detachment.

d) Potential for acute angle-closure glaucoma.

9. Which laboratory test would be most appropriate for monitoring anticoagulation therapy in a patient on warfarin with atrial fibrillation?

a) PT/INR.

b) aPTT.

c) CBC.

d) CMP.

10. How should an optometrist manage a patient presenting with jaundice, high ALT, AST, and bilirubin levels, and a history of chronic alcohol use?

a) Recommend liver detox supplements.

b) Refer to hepatology for further evaluation and management.

c) Prescribe antivirals for hepatitis.

d) Suggest lifestyle changes and monitor liver function tests.

11. What is the clinical relevance of a positive HLA-B27 test in a patient with recurrent anterior uveitis and back pain?

a) Suggests a high likelihood of ankylosing spondylitis.

b) Indicates systemic lupus erythematosus.

c) Reflects rheumatoid arthritis.

d) Points to multiple sclerosis.

12. When should an optometrist order an MRI with the FIESTA protocol, and what specific pathology might this help identify?

a) For patients with suspected optic neuritis to visualize nerve inflammation.

b) For patients with trigeminal neuralgia to detect vascular compression.

c) For patients with diabetic retinopathy to assess retinal changes.

d) For patients with suspected brain masses.

13. In a patient with suspected thyroid dysfunction, what combination of TFT results would indicate primary hypothyroidism?

a) High TSH, low Free T4, low Free T3.

b) Low TSH, high Free T4, high Free T3.

c) Normal TSH, low Free T4, low Free T3.

d) High TSH, high Free T4, low Free T3.

14. What imaging modality and findings would be most indicative of carotid artery stenosis in a patient with transient ischemic attacks (TIA)?

a) Carotid duplex ultrasound showing increased blood flow velocity.

b) MRI showing white matter lesions.

c) CT scan showing brain atrophy.

d) X-ray showing calcified plaques.

15. What clinical condition is suggested by prolonged aPTT and normal PT in a patient with spontaneous bruising and bleeding?

a) Hemophilia.

b) Vitamin K deficiency.

c) Hypercoagulable state.

d) Liver cirrhosis.

16. How should an optometrist handle a situation where a radiology report and clinical findings do not align in a patient with persistent headaches and visual disturbances?

a) Trust the radiology report and ignore clinical symptoms.

b) Request a re-evaluation or second opinion from radiology.

c) Discharge the patient with reassurance.

d) Prescribe pain relief medication and monitor.

17. **What is the significance of finding a high platelet count in a CBC in a patient presenting with visual disturbances and headaches?**

a) Indicates possible chronic myeloproliferative disorder.

b) Suggests iron deficiency anemia.

c) Reflects dehydration.

d) Points to liver dysfunction.

18. **Which diagnostic test is necessary for evaluating a patient with suspected temporal arteritis presenting with headache, jaw claudication, and vision changes?**

a) Erythrocyte Sedimentation Rate (ESR).

b) Fasting Blood Glucose.

c) Lipid Profile.

d) Comprehensive Metabolic Profile (CMP).

19. **What would be the most appropriate next step for an optometrist if a patient's CMP results**

indicate significantly elevated creatinine and BUN levels?

a) Advise increased water intake and repeat the test.

b) Refer to nephrology for further evaluation of potential kidney dysfunction.

c) Suggest dietary changes to lower protein intake.

d) Prescribe diuretics to reduce BUN levels.

20. **Why is it essential for an optometrist to understand the implications of lab and imaging results even if they are not the primary interpreters of these diagnostics?**

a) To ensure they can effectively integrate these findings into the overall management plan for their patients.

b) To independently diagnose conditions without consulting specialists.

c) To reduce the need for referrals to other healthcare professionals.

d) To avoid discussing results with patients directly.

Answers

Answers

1. b) Indicates inflammatory or autoimmune etiology; refer to rheumatology.

- **Rationale**: Persistent high ESR with recurrent uveitis suggests a systemic inflammatory or autoimmune condition, warranting referral to a rheumatologist.

2. b) Refer urgently to hematology/oncology for suspected acute leukemia.

- **Rationale**: A high WBC count with blasts indicates acute leukemia, requiring immediate hematology/oncology referral.

3. c) Assess mean corpuscular volume (MCV) and red cell distribution width (RDW).

- **Rationale**: Chronic disease anemia typically

presents with normal MCV and RDW, while iron deficiency anemia shows low MCV and high RDW.

4. **a) Assessing for carotid artery stenosis or intracranial aneurysms.**

• **Rationale**: CTA is used to evaluate vascular abnormalities like carotid stenosis and aneurysms in patients with visual field defects and stroke symptoms.

5. **b) MRI showing periventricular white matter lesions.**

• **Rationale**: MRI with periventricular white matter lesions is indicative of multiple sclerosis.

6. **b) Suggests a non-specific inflammatory response; further evaluation needed.**

• **Rationale**: High CRP with normal ESR suggests acute inflammation, requiring further investigation to identify the cause.

7. **c) Speckled pattern alone cannot differentiate; clinical correlation is essential.**

• **Rationale**: A speckled ANA pattern can be seen in various autoimmune diseases, requiring clinical correlation for accurate diagnosis.

8. **a) Risk of diabetic retinopathy and macular edema.**

• **Rationale**: Poorly controlled diabetes with high blood glucose and HbA1c increases the risk of diabetic retinopathy and macular edema, leading to fluctuating vision.

9. a) PT/INR.

• **Rationale**: PT/INR is used to monitor anticoagulation therapy in patients on warfarin, ensuring they remain within the therapeutic range.

10. b) Refer to hepatology for further evaluation and management.

• **Rationale**: Elevated liver enzymes and bilirubin in a patient with chronic alcohol use indicate possible liver disease, requiring hepatology referral.

11. a) Suggests a high likelihood of ankylosing spondylitis.

• **Rationale**: HLA-B27 is associated with ankylosing spondylitis, especially in patients with recurrent anterior uveitis and back pain.

12. b) For patients with trigeminal neuralgia to detect vascular compression.

• **Rationale**: FIESTA MRI is excellent for visualizing cranial nerve lesions, including vascular compression in trigeminal neuralgia.

13. a) High TSH, low Free T4, low Free T3.

• **Rationale**: This combination of thyroid function tests indicates primary hypothyroidism due to thyroid gland dysfunction.

14. **a) Carotid duplex ultrasound showing increased blood flow velocity.**

• **Rationale**: Carotid duplex ultrasound can detect increased blood flow velocity due to stenosis, making it essential for assessing carotid artery disease.

15. **a) Hemophilia.**

• **Rationale**: Prolonged aPTT with normal PT suggests a deficiency in intrinsic clotting factors, characteristic of hemophilia.

16. **b) Request a re-evaluation or second opinion from radiology.**

• **Rationale**: Discrepancies between clinical findings and radiology reports should prompt a re-evaluation to ensure accurate diagnosis and management.

17. **a) Indicates possible chronic myeloproliferative disorder.**

• **Rationale**: A high platelet count can indicate chronic myeloproliferative disorders, which may present with visual disturbances and headaches.

18. **a) Erythrocyte Sedimentation Rate (ESR).**

• **Rationale**: High ESR in a patient with symptoms of temporal arteritis supports the diagnosis and necessitates urgent treatment to prevent vision loss.

19. **b) Refer to nephrology for further evaluation of potential kidney dysfunction.**

• **Rationale**: Elevated creatinine and BUN levels indicate possible kidney dysfunction, requiring nephrology referral for further assessment.

20. a) To ensure they can effectively integrate these findings into the overall management plan for their patients.

• **Rationale**: Understanding lab and imaging results allows optometrists to make informed decisions and provide comprehensive patient care, even if they are not the primary interpreters of these diagnostics.

About the Author

With 27 years on the private practice front lines as an optometric physician prior to earning his MD, Dr. Martinelli brings years of extensive clinical experience, combined with medicine, providing rare insight and guidance in the art of patient management.

He offers not theory, but high-yield clinical knowledge to help build the practice you deserve simply by taking proper care of people, who also happen to be your patients.

Dr. Martinelli is a graduate of St. George's University School of Medicine, Pennsylvania College of Optometry, and Washington & Jefferson College. He is a physician member of the American Medical Association (AMA), American Optometric Association (AOA), and Fellow of the American Academy of Optometry (FAAO).

His clinical articles have been featured over the years in various publications. He very much enjoys teaching, and for more than a decade taught countless students in his practice as a preceptor in ocular disease for the Pennsylvania College of Optometry.

Dr. Martinelli has spoken for Alcon and Allergan, as well as nationally and internationally with topics involving medical eye care, glaucoma, and refractive surgery such as LASIK.

He continues to actively see patients daily in private practice.

Ophthalmic Physician Website

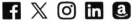